WHEAT ALLERGY

THE TIPS FOR TREATING WHEAT ALLERGY

DR. KATE .P

Contents

CHAPTER ONE 3

INTRODUCTION 3

Symptoms 4

An allergic reaction 5

When to visit a physician 6

Reasons 7

Wheat protein sources...7

RISK ELEMENTS 11

Getting Ready for Your Consultation 12

What you're capable of...12

What to anticipate from your physician 14

Exams and diagnosis 15

CHAPTER TWO 16

MEDICATIONS AND SUBTLES 18

Medications 18

Emergency medical attention 19

WAY OF LIFE AND DOMESTIC MEDICINE 20

THE END 23

CHAPTER ONE

INTRODUCTION

One of the top eight food allergies in the US is wheat allergy, which is an allergic reaction to meals containing wheat. Eating wheat and, under certain situations, breathing wheat flour might cause allergic responses. Numerous foods, even those you might not think about, like beer, soy sauce, and ketchup, contain wheat.

The main treatment for wheat allergy is to avoid wheat. Should you unintentionally consume wheat, you may need to take medication to control allergic responses.

Although both disorders are different, wheat allergy and celiac disease are commonly mistaken. An allergy to wheat proteins results in an antibody that triggers the allergy. Gluten, a specific wheat protein, triggers an aberrant immune response in those who have celiac disease.

Symptoms

After consuming anything that contains wheat, a kid or adult with a wheat allergy is likely to have symptoms minutes to hours later. Symptoms of a wheat allergy include:

mouth or throat swelling, stinging, or irritation

Itchy rash, hives, or skin swelling

congestion in the nose

Headache

eyes that are wet and itchy

breathing difficulties

nausea, vomiting, or cramping

The diarrhea

An allergic reaction

By the time they are three to five years old, the majority of young children who have wheat allergy have outgrown it.

An allergic reaction

Some people may get anaphylaxis, a potentially fatal reaction, from a wheat allergy. Besides the usual indications and symptoms of wheat allergy, anaphylaxis can result in:

throat swelling or constriction

Tightness or pain in the chest

severe respiratory difficulties

difficulty swallowing

pale, azure complexion

lightheadedness or fainting

rapid heart rate

When to visit a physician

Anaphylaxis symptoms should be reported by calling 911 or your local emergency number. A medical emergency that needs to be treated right away is anaphylaxis.

Consult your physician if you think you or your kid may be allergic to wheat or any other food.

Reasons

Exposure to a wheat protein primes your immune system for an allergic reaction if you have a wheat allergy. Any one of the four groups of wheat proteins gliadin, albumin, globulin, and gluten can cause an allergy.

Wheat protein sources

While some sources of wheat proteins, like bread, are evident, many prepared foods contain wheat proteins, and gluten in particular. Some cosmetics, bath treatments, and play dough also contain wheat proteins. Wheat proteins can be found in the following foods:

Breadstuffs and breadcrumbs

Muffins and cakes

Cookies

cereals for breakfast

Pasta

couscous

Farina

Semolina

Spelt

Crackers

lager

vegetable protein hydrolyzed

Soy sauce

Certain condiments, like ketchup

Meat products, such cold cuts and hot dogs

dairy goods, like ice cream

organic flavorings

starch that has gelatinized

altered food starch

Gum made with vegetables

Licorice

Jelly beans

Hard candies

Although the likelihood is low, if you have a wheat allergy, you may also be allergic to barley, oats, and rye. A wheat-free diet is less restrictive than a gluten-free diet if you're not sensitive to cereals other than wheat.

Anaphylaxis brought on by exercise and wheat dependence

Some wheat allergy sufferers only experience symptoms if they exercise shortly after consuming wheat. Your body's altered state brought on by exercise can exacerbate an immune system reaction to wheat proteins or cause an allergic reaction. Usually, this disease causes anaphylaxis, which can be fatal.

RISK ELEMENTS

A few things could make you more susceptible to getting a wheat allergy:

background in the family. If either or both of your parents suffer from hay fever or other allergies, you have a higher chance of developing a wheat allergy or any other type of allergy.

Years old. Due to their developing immune and digestive systems, newborns and toddlers are most commonly affected by wheat allergy. Wheat allergy is often outgrown by children, but it can also strike adults, usually as a cross-sensitivity to grass pollen.

Getting Ready for Your Consultation

If you think you or your child may have a wheat allergy or another allergy, get in to see your doctor. Make an appointment with your pediatrician or family physician for diagnostic testing; they could recommend that you see an allergist for certain conditions.

What you're capable of

Make a list of the following items for your doctor to have ready for your visit:

symptoms, including those that don't seem to be connected to an allergy

The history of allergies and asthma in your family, particularly the presence of particular allergies

vitamins, minerals, or other dietary supplements that you or your kid take

Include a list of inquiries for your physician, such as:

Are allergies most likely the cause of the symptoms?

Do I require allergy testing?

Do I need to visit an allergist?

Does carrying epinephrine around in case of anaphylaxis make sense?

Do you possess any printed materials, such as brochures? Which websites would you suggest?

Do not be afraid to ask additional questions.

What to anticipate from your physician

You will probably be asked a lot of questions by your doctor, such as:

When do symptoms start to show up after eating?

Do symptoms appear to be connected to a particular food?

What solid meals does your infant consume, if any?

Has your baby's diet recently included any new foods?

Has anyone else get ill after consuming the same food?

To what extent was a meal suspected of causing an allergy consumed?

What other items were consumed concurrently or shortly afterward?

Exams and diagnosis

Your doctor will use a physical examination, a thorough medical history, and certain tests to assist reach a diagnosis. Among the tests or diagnostic instruments are:

CHAPTER TWO

Skin test. On your upper back or forearm, tiny drops of pure allergen extracts, including wheat protein extracts, are pricked into the surface of your skin. Your doctor or nurse checks for allergic response symptoms after 15 minutes.

You might be allergic to wheat if you get a red, itchy lump where the wheat protein extract was prickly applied to your skin. Itching and redness are the most frequent side effects of these skin examinations.

blood examination. In case a skin ailment or potential medication interactions hinder your ability to undergo a skin test, your physician can recommend a blood test that looks for certain antibodies that cause allergies to common allergens, such as wheat proteins.

food journal. For a while, your doctor might urge you to keep a thorough journal of everything you eat, when you eat it, and when you start experiencing symptoms.

diet of elimination. Your physician can advise you to cut out specific foods from your diet, especially if they are common allergies. You will progressively resume eating meals as directed by your doctor, and you will record the return of symptoms.

testing of food challenges. As you watch for allergy symptoms, you consume amounts of food that may be the cause of your allergy. You start with a modest amount of the food and progressively increase your intake while being watched.

MEDICATIONS AND SUBTLES

The best treatment for wheat allergy is to avoid wheat proteins. Read product labels carefully because so many prepared foods contain wheat proteins.

Medications

Antihistamines have the potential to lessen wheat allergy symptoms and indications. After being exposed to wheat, you can use these medications to help manage your reaction and ease your discomfort. Find out from your doctor if you should take an over-the-counter or prescription allergy medication.

Anaphylaxis can be treated urgently with epinephrine. You may need to always have two injectable doses of epinephrine on hand if you're susceptible to a severe reaction to wheat. For those with a high risk of potentially fatal anaphylaxis, it is advised to carry a backup pen in case symptoms worsen before help arrives.

Emergency medical attention

Even after an adrenaline injection, emergency medical attention is crucial for anyone experiencing an allergic reaction to wheat. As soon as you can, dial your local emergency number or 911.

If you are unintentionally exposed to wheat, you can take precautions to prevent exposure to wheat proteins and make sure you receive treatment right away.

Inform others as needed. If your child has a wheat allergy, make sure that everyone who looks after them, such as the school nurse, principal, and instructors, is aware of the allergy and the symptoms of wheat exposure. Make sure school staff members are aware of how to use an epipen, if needed, and that they should call emergency services right away if your child has one. Notify friends, family, and coworkers about your personal food allergy.

Put on a bracelet. If you suffer anaphylaxis and are unable to communicate, a medical identification bracelet that details the allergy and the need for emergency care can be helpful.

Read labels at all times. Before you read the label, don't assume that a product is free of anything you can't eat. Gluten and other wheat proteins are utilized as food thickeners and can be found in a variety of surprising places. Additionally, you shouldn't assume that a product is always safe just because you've used a particular brand. Ingredients are interchangeable.

Purchase gluten-free products. Foods that are gluten-free and safe for those with wheat allergies can be found in certain specialty shops and supermarkets. But, they might also be devoid of grains that you can consume, so limiting your diet to only gluten-free items might be pointless.

Consult cookbooks that are wheat-free. You can enjoy baked goods and other dishes produced with wheat substitutes and cook more safely if you use cookbooks that specialize in recipes without wheat.

Eat outside with caution. Inform the staff of the severity of your allergy if you eat anything that contains wheat. Get simple recipes made using fresh ingredients. Steer clear of deep-fried items that may have been cooked with other wheat-containing foods or sauces that could include hidden sources of wheat proteins.

THE END